CARNIVORE

DIET COOKBOOK FOR WOMEN

50 Yummy, Protein-Rich Animal-Based Recipes that Support Optimal Health, Hormonal Balance, and Vitality in Women

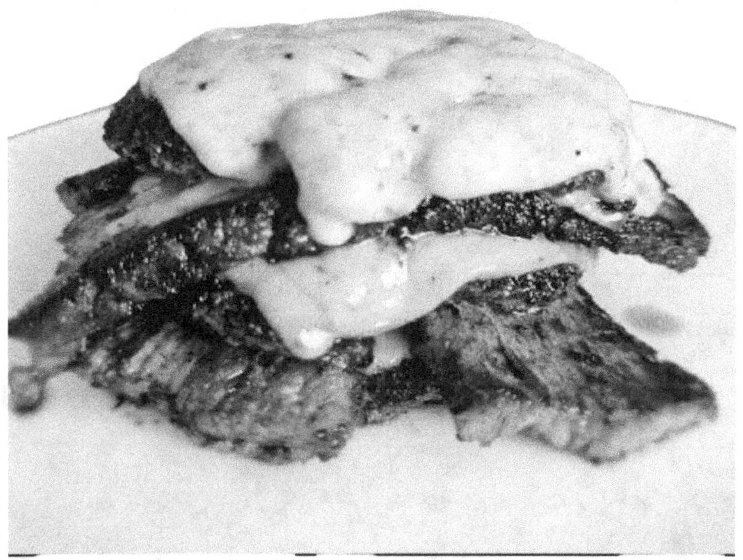

DR. COLE HULL

COPYRIGHT

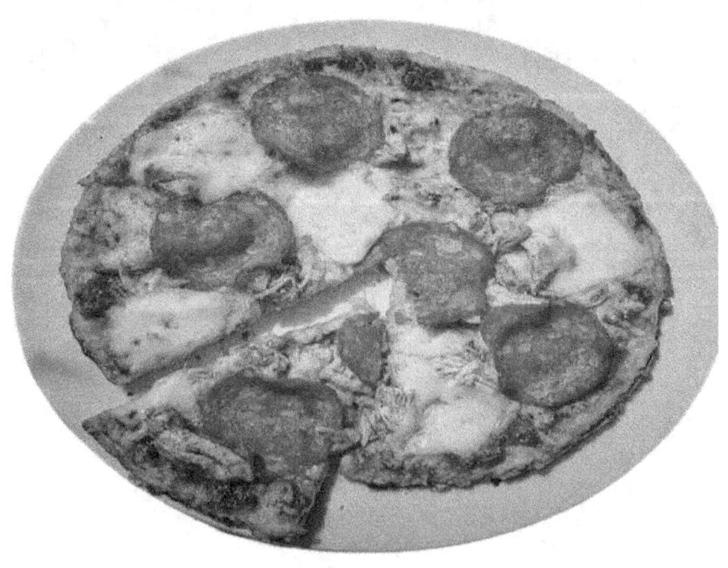

TABLE OF CONTENT

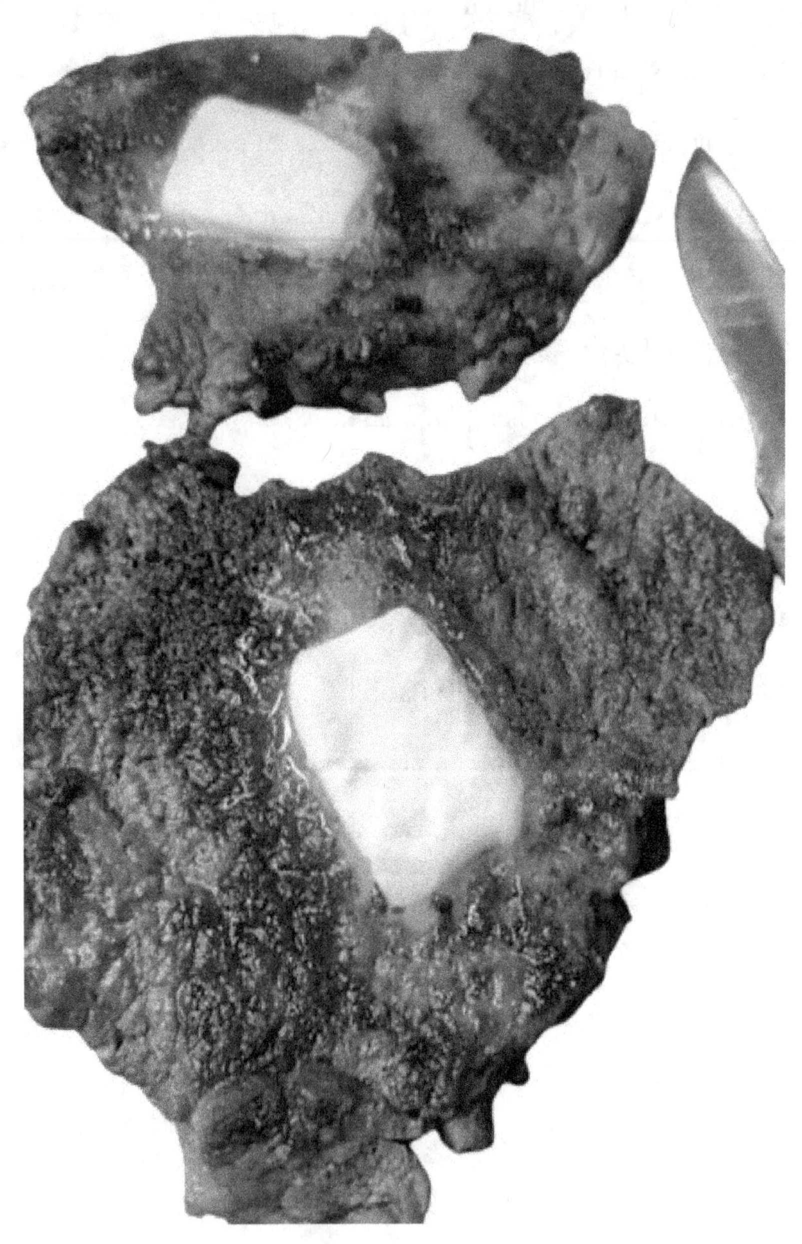

1. INTRODUCTION

Welcome to the "Carnivore Diet Cookbook for Women," a culinary adventure designed for women who want to discover the incredible health advantages of a carnivorous lifestyle. For women, it's important to recognize and address our specific nutritional requirements in order to maintain optimal health. This cookbook goes beyond being a mere compilation of recipes; it's a tribute to a way of life that has had a profound impact on countless individuals.

Starting a carnivore diet can have a significant impact on women's health. It's not only about simplifying eating habits, but also about embracing a traditional approach to nourishing our bodies with nutritious, animal-based foods. This diet emphasizes the importance of ingredients that are high in protein, rich in healthy fats, and low in carbohydrates. The goal is to ensure you're getting all the essential nutrients for optimal health, hormonal balance, and overall vitality.

The recipes in this cookbook are thoughtfully created, focusing on both their nutritional value and delicious taste, while also being easy to follow. Our recipes are unique, creative, and varied, guaranteeing that your carnivore diet experience is never boring.

With a wide range of delicious recipes, you'll discover a variety of dishes that are not only tasty but also promote a healthy lifestyle. These recipes have been enjoyed by many women who have experienced the positive impact they can have on both their physical and mental well-being.

This cookbook is tailored for the modern woman who prioritizes health while juggling a busy lifestyle. Whether you're an experienced cook or a beginner in the kitchen, these recipes are designed to be easy to follow, time-saving, and delicious. They go beyond being mere dishes; they serve as a tribute to the resilience and energy of women who opt to nourish their bodies in a manner aligned with nature's intentions.

So, let's start this adventure together. Discover the incredible benefits of a carnivore diet and how it can revolutionize your meals, as well as improve your overall health and well-being. Welcome to the "Carnivore Diet Cookbook for Women"–your go-to resource for achieving a stronger and healthier version of yourself.

2. YUMMY MEAT-BASED DIET RECIPES FOR WOMEN

1. Classic Beef Steak

Prep Time: 5 minutes
Cook Time: 10 minutes

Ingredients:

- 1 8-oz beef steak (ribeye or sirloin)
- Salt to taste

Preparation Instructions:

1. Preheat your skillet over high heat.

2. Season the steak generously with salt.

3. Place the steak in the skillet and cook for 4-5 minutes per side for medium-rare.

4. Let the steak rest for 5 minutes before slicing.

Health Benefit:

High in protein and iron, supporting muscle maintenance and energy levels.

2. Crispy Chicken Thighs

Prep Time: 5 minutes

Cook Time: 35 minutes

Ingredients:

  - 4 chicken thighs, skin-on
  - Salt to taste

Preparation Instructions:

  1. Preheat the oven to 400°F (200°C).

  2. Season chicken thighs with salt on both sides.

  3. Place skin-side up on a baking sheet and bake for 35 minutes, until the skin is crispy.

  4. Let rest for 5 minutes before serving.

Health Benefit:

Rich in selenium and B vitamins, supporting thyroid function and energy metabolism.

3. Baked Pork Chops

Prep Time: 5 minutes

Cook Time: 25 minutes

Ingredients:

  - 2 pork chops, 1-inch thick

  - Salt to taste

Preparation Instructions:

  1. Preheat oven to 375°F (190°C).

  2. Season pork chops with salt.

  3. Bake for 25 minutes, or until the internal temperature reaches 145°F (63°C).

  4. Rest for 3 minutes before serving.

Health Benefit:

Good source of B vitamins and zinc, important for brain health and immune function.

4. Seared Lamb Ribs

Prep Time: 5 minutes
Cook Time: 15 minutes

Ingredients:

  - 4 lamb ribs
  - Salt to taste

Preparation Instructions:

  1. Season lamb ribs with salt.
  2. Heat a skillet over medium-high heat and sear ribs for about 3-4 minutes per side.
  3. Let rest for 5 minutes, then serve.

Health Benefit:

Lamb is a great source of high-quality protein and iron, beneficial for muscle repair and oxygen transport in the blood.

5. Homemade Beef Jerky

Prep Time: 15 minutes (plus marinating time)
Cook Time: 3-4 hours

Ingredients:

- 1 lb lean beef (top round), thinly sliced
- Salt to taste

Preparation Instructions:

1. Season beef slices with salt.
2. Arrange slices on a baking rack over a baking sheet.
3. Bake at a low temperature (175°F or 80°C) for 3-4 hours, until dry and leathery.
4. Store in an airtight container.

Health Benefit:

High in protein and low in fat, making it a great snack to support lean muscle mass.

6. Salmon Sashimi

Prep Time: 10 minutes
Cook Time: 0 minutes
Ingredients:

  - 8 oz fresh salmon fillet, sashimi-grade
  - Salt (optional)

Preparation Instructions:

  1. Slice the salmon fillet against the grain into thin slices.
  2. Arrange on a plate and sprinkle with a tiny amount of salt if desired.
  3. Serve immediately.

Health Benefit: Rich in omega-3 fatty acids, supporting cardiovascular health and reducing inflammation.

7. Chicken Liver Pâté

Prep Time: 10 minutes
Cook Time: 15 minutes
Ingredients:

  - 1 lb chicken livers, cleaned
  - 1/2 cup butter
  - Salt to taste

Preparation Instructions:

1. Melt half the butter in a pan and cook the livers until just done.

2. Blend livers with remaining butter and salt until smooth.

3. Chill in the fridge until set.

Health Benefit: High in B12 and iron, essential for red blood cell formation and cognitive function.

8. Bacon and Egg Frittata

Prep Time: 5 minutes

Cook Time: 15 minutes

Ingredients:

- 6 eggs

- 4 slices of bacon, chopped

- Salt to taste

Preparation Instructions:

1. Preheat the oven to 350°F (175°C).

2. Cook bacon in an oven-proof skillet until crisp. Drain excess fat.

3. Beat eggs with salt, pour over bacon in the skillet.

4. Bake for 15 minutes or until eggs are set.

Health Benefit: Eggs and bacon provide a high-quality protein source for muscle maintenance and repair.

9. Grilled Ribeye Steak

Prep Time: 5 minutes
Cook Time: 10 minutes

Ingredients:
  - 1 8-oz ribeye steak
  - Salt to taste

Preparation Instructions:
  1. Preheat grill to high heat.
  2. Season steak with salt.
  3. Grill for 4-5 minutes per side for medium-rare.
  4. Let rest for 5 minutes, then serve.

Health Benefit:
A good source of creatine and iron, supporting energy production and muscle function.

10. Pork Belly

Prep Time: 5 minutes

Cook Time: 3 hours

Ingredients:

- 1 lb pork belly, skin-on
- Salt to taste

Preparation Instructions:

1. Score the pork belly skin and season with salt.
2. Roast at 275°F (135°C) for 2.5 hours.
3. Increase the oven temperature to 400°F (200°C) for the last 30 minutes to crisp the skin.
4. Let rest, then slice and serve.

Health Benefit:

Pork belly is calorie-dense and high in B vitamins, providing energy and supporting metabolic processes.

11. Beef Bone Broth

Prep Time: 10 minutes
Cook Time: 24 hours

Ingredients:

  - 2 lbs beef bones

  - Water to cover

  - Salt to taste

Preparation Instructions:

1. Place beef bones in a large pot and cover with water. Add salt.

2. Bring to a boil, then reduce heat and simmer gently for 24 hours, adding water as needed to keep bones covered.

3. Strain the broth and cool. Skim off fat that solidifies on top if desired.

Health Benefit:

Rich in collagen and minerals, supporting joint health and skin elasticity.

12. Butter-Poached Fish

Prep Time: 5 minutes

Cook Time: 10 minutes

Ingredients:

- 2 fish fillets (e.g., cod or salmon)
- 1/4 cup butter
- Salt to taste

Preparation Instructions:

1. In a skillet, melt butter over low heat.
2. Add the fish fillets and cook gently for 4-5 minutes per side, spooning butter over them as they cook.
3. Serve immediately.

Health Benefit:

Provides omega-3 fatty acids and lean protein, supporting heart health and muscle maintenance.

13. Bacon Roses

Prep Time: 15 minutes
Cook Time: 20 minutes
Ingredients:

- 12 slices of bacon

Preparation Instructions:

1. Roll each bacon slice into a tight spiral to resemble a rosebud.
2. Place each bacon rosebud into a muffin tin compartment.
3. Bake at 375°F (190°C) for 20-25 minutes until crisp.
4. Allow to cool slightly before removing from the tin.

Health Benefit: Bacon provides a good source of fat and protein, which can help to sustain energy levels.

14. Scrambled Eggs with Cheese

Prep Time: 2 minutes
Cook Time: 5 minutes
Ingredients:

- 4 eggs
- 1/4 cup shredded cheese (e.g., cheddar)
- 1 tablespoon butter
- Salt to taste

Preparation Instructions:

1. Beat the eggs with salt.

2. Melt butter in a pan over medium heat, add the eggs, and cook, stirring gently.

3. When the eggs start to set, sprinkle cheese over them and continue to cook until the cheese melts and eggs are cooked to your liking.

Health Benefit: Eggs and cheese are high in calcium and protein, supporting bone health and muscle function.

15. Duck Breast

Prep Time: 5 minutes
Cook Time: 15 minutes
Ingredients:

- 2 duck breasts, skin on
- Salt to taste

Preparation Instructions:

1. Score the duck skin in a diamond pattern and season with salt.

2. Place skin-side down in a cold skillet, then turn heat to medium. Cook until the skin is crisp, about 6-8 minutes.

3. Flip the breasts over and cook for another 4-7 minutes for medium-rare.

4. Let rest before slicing.

Health Benefit: Duck is a good source of B vitamins and iron, which are important for energy metabolism and blood health.

16. Crispy Chicken Skins

Prep Time: 5 minutes
Cook Time: 15 minutes
Ingredients:
  - Chicken skins from 4 thighs
  - Salt to taste

Preparation Instructions:
  1. Preheat oven to 400°F (200°C).
  2. Lay chicken skins flat on a baking sheet, season with salt.
  3. Bake for 15 minutes, or until golden and crisp.

Health Benefit:
Provides a source of collagen and fat, which can contribute to skin health and satiety.

17. Roasted Turkey Legs

Prep Time: 5 minutes

Cook Time: 1 hour 30 minutes

Ingredients:

- 2 turkey legs
- Salt to taste

Preparation Instructions:

1. Preheat oven to 350°F (175°C).
2. Season turkey legs with salt and place in a roasting pan.
3. Roast for 1.5 hours, or until the internal temperature reaches 165°F (74°C).

Health Benefit: Turkey is lean protein, supporting muscle maintenance and satiety without high fat content.

18. Slow-Cooked Beef Brisket

Prep Time: 5 minutes

Cook Time: 8 hours

Ingredients:

- 3 lb beef brisket
- Salt to taste

Preparation Instructions:

1. Season the brisket generously with salt.

2. Place in a slow cooker and cook on low for 8 hours or until tender.

3. Slice against the grain and serve.

Health Benefit: Brisket is rich in proteins and minerals like iron and zinc, supporting immune function and muscle growth.

19. Pan-Fried Fish Fillets

Prep Time: 5 minutes

Cook Time: 10 minutes

Ingredients:

- 2 fish fillets (e.g., tilapia, cod)
- 2 tablespoons animal fat (e.g., lard, tallow)
- Salt to taste

Preparation Instructions:

1. Season fish fillets with salt.

2. Heat fat in a pan over medium-high heat and fry the fillets for about 4-5 minutes per side, until cooked through.

Health Benefit: Fish is a great source of lean protein and omega-3 fatty acids, beneficial for heart and brain health.

20. Bacon-Wrapped Asparagus

Prep Time: 10 minutes

Cook Time: 20 minutes

Ingredients:

- 12 asparagus spears

- 6 slices of bacon, cut in half

Preparation Instructions:

1. Wrap a piece of bacon around each asparagus spear.

2. Place on a baking sheet and bake at 400°F (200°C) for 20 minutes, or until the bacon is crispy.

Health Benefit: While asparagus is a vegetable and not strictly carnivore, this dish could be an exception for those who occasionally include high-nutrient, low-carb veggies. Asparagus provides fiber, vitamins, and minerals, supporting digestive health and nutrient absorption.

For those strictly adhering to a 100% carnivore diet, you can replace asparagus with another suitable animal-based ingredient, such as cheese sticks or sausage links.

21. Carnivore Meatballs

Prep Time: 10 minutes

Cook Time: 20 minutes

Ingredients:

- 1 lb ground beef
- 1 egg
- Salt to taste

Preparation Instructions:

1. Preheat your oven to 375°F (190°C).
2. Mix ground beef, egg, and salt thoroughly.
3. Form into 1-inch balls and place on a baking sheet.
4. Bake for 20 minutes or until cooked through.

Health Benefit:

Provides a high amount of protein and B vitamins, essential for energy metabolism and maintaining muscle mass.

22. Butter-Basted Chicken Breast

Prep Time: 5 minutes

Cook Time: 15 minutes

Ingredients:

  - 2 chicken breasts

  - 2 tablespoons butter

  - Salt to taste

Preparation Instructions:

1. Season chicken breasts with salt.

2. Melt butter in a skillet over medium heat, add chicken and cook for 7 minutes on one side.

3. Flip, then spoon melted butter over the chicken for another 7-8 minutes or until fully cooked.

Health Benefit:

Chicken is a lean protein source that supports muscle repair and maintenance, while butter adds beneficial fats for hormone production.

23. Baked Ham

Prep Time: 5 minutes

Cook Time: 2 hours

Ingredients:

  - 1 whole ham, pre-cooked

  - Salt to taste

Preparation Instructions:

  1. Preheat oven to 325°F (165°C).

  2. Place ham in a roasting pan and season with salt.

  3. Bake for about 2 hours or until heated through.

Health Benefit: Ham provides a good source of protein, B vitamins, and minerals like zinc, supporting immune health and energy levels.

24. Crispy Pork Rinds

Prep Time: 5 minutes

Cook Time: 3 hours

Ingredients:

  - Pork skin, cut into strips

  - Salt to taste

Preparation Instructions:

1. Preheat your oven to 250°F (120°C).

2. Place pork skin strips on a baking rack over a baking sheet, season with salt.

3. Bake for about 3 hours or until crispy.

Health Benefit: Pork rinds are a zero-carb snack, high in fat and protein, which can help maintain satiety and support a ketogenic metabolic state.

25. Beef Liver Fried in Bacon Fat

Prep Time: 5 minutes

Cook Time: 10 minutes

Ingredients:

- 1 lb beef liver, sliced

- 2 tablespoons bacon fat

- Salt to taste

Preparation Instructions:

1. Heat bacon fat in a skillet over medium heat.

2. Season liver slices with salt and fry for about 3-5 minutes per side.

3. Serve hot.

Health Benefit:

Liver is one of the most nutrient-dense foods, rich in vitamin A, iron, and B vitamins, supporting skin health, energy production, and cognitive function.

26. Grilled Sardines

Prep Time: 5 minutes
Cook Time: 10 minutes
Ingredients:

- 1 lb fresh sardines, cleaned
- Salt to taste

Preparation Instructions:
  1. Preheat grill to medium-high heat.
  2. Season sardines with salt and place on the grill.
  3. Grill for about 5 minutes per side or until cooked through.

Health Benefit:

Sardines are an excellent source of omega-3 fatty acids, vitamin D, and calcium, supporting cardiovascular health, bone density, and immune function.

27. Roasted Bone Marrow

Prep Time: 5 minutes

Cook Time: 20 minutes

Ingredients:

- 4 beef marrow bones, cut lengthwise

- Salt to taste

Preparation Instructions:

1. Preheat oven to 450°F (230°C).

2. Place marrow bones on a baking sheet, season with salt.

3. Roast for 20 minutes or until marrow is soft and slightly bubbly.

Health Benefit: Bone marrow is rich in healthy fats, collagen, and other nutrients that support joint health, immune function, and skin health.

28. Egg Muffins with Ham

Prep Time: 10 minutes

Cook Time: 20 minutes

Ingredients:

- 6 eggs

- 1/2 cup diced ham

- Salt to taste

Preparation Instructions:

1. Preheat oven to 350°F (175°C).

2. Whisk eggs and salt together, stir in diced ham.

3. Pour into muffin tins and bake for 20 minutes or until set.

Health Benefit: Eggs provide high-quality protein and nutrients like choline, which supports brain health. Ham adds additional protein and flavor.

29. Pork Sausage Patties

Prep Time: 10 minutes
Cook Time: 10 minutes
Ingredients:

- 1 lb ground pork
- Salt and black pepper to taste

Preparation Instructions:

1. Season ground pork with salt and pepper, and form into patties.

2. Cook in a skillet over medium heat for about 5 minutes per side or until cooked through.

Health Benefit: Pork is a good source of thiamin, which is essential for energy metabolism and nerve function.

30. Omelette with Goat Cheese

Prep Time: 5 minutes

Cook Time: 5 minutes

Ingredients:

- 3 eggs

- 1/4 cup crumbled goat cheese

- Salt to taste

Preparation Instructions:

1. Beat eggs with salt.
2. Pour into a hot, buttered skillet, and cook until the bottom sets.
3. Sprinkle goat cheese over half the omelette, fold, and serve.

Health Benefit: Offers a high-quality protein source and is rich in vitamins A and D, as well as calcium, which are important for bone health and immune function.

31. Bison Burger

Prep Time: 5 minutes

Cook Time: 10 minutes

Ingredients:

- 1 lb ground bison

- Salt to taste

Preparation Instructions:

1. Preheat your grill or skillet over medium-high heat.

2. Form the ground bison into 4 patties and season with salt.

3. Grill or pan-fry for about 5 minutes per side for medium doneness.

4. Let the burgers rest for a few minutes before serving.

Health Benefit: Bison meat is leaner than beef and provides high-quality protein, iron, and B vitamins, which are essential for energy metabolism and muscle maintenance.

32. Venison Steaks

Prep Time: 5 minutes

Cook Time: 6 minutes

Ingredients:

- 2 venison steaks, about 6 oz each
- Salt to taste

Preparation Instructions:

1. Preheat a skillet or grill to high heat.

2. Season venison steaks with salt.

3. Cook for 3 minutes per side for medium-rare, or longer to your desired doneness.

4. Let the steaks rest for a few minutes before serving.

Health Benefit: Venison is a great source of lean protein and is rich in iron, which is crucial for oxygen transport and energy levels, making it beneficial for women's health.

33. Bacon-Wrapped Shrimp

Prep Time: 10 minutes
Cook Time: 15 minutes
Ingredients:

- 12 large shrimp, peeled and deveined
- 6 bacon strips, cut in half
- Salt to taste

Preparation Instructions:

1. Preheat your oven to 400°F (200°C).
2. Wrap each shrimp with a half strip of bacon and secure with a toothpick.
3. Season lightly with salt and place on a baking sheet.
4. Bake for 15 minutes, or until bacon is crispy and shrimp is pink.

Health Benefit: Shrimp is high in protein and iodine, which is essential for thyroid function, while bacon adds a satisfying source of fat.

34. Smoked Trout

Prep Time: 5 minutes

Cook Time: 2 hours

Ingredients:

- 2 whole trout, cleaned
- Salt to taste

Preparation Instructions:

1. Preheat your smoker to 225°F (107°C).

2. Season the trout inside and out with salt.

3. Smoke for about 2 hours, or until the fish flakes easily with a fork.

Health Benefit: Trout is rich in omega-3 fatty acids, which are beneficial for heart health and reducing inflammation.

35. Carnivore "Pizza"

Prep Time: 15 minutes

Cook Time: 20 minutes

Ingredients:

- 1 lb ground chicken (for crust)
- 1 cup shredded mozzarella cheese

- 4 oz pepperoni slices

- Salt to taste

Preparation Instructions:

1. Preheat your oven to 400°F (200°C).

2. Press the ground chicken onto a baking sheet lined with parchment paper, forming a thin layer for the crust. Season with salt.

3. Bake the crust for 10 minutes, then remove from the oven.

4. Sprinkle the mozzarella over the crust and top with pepperoni slices.

5. Return to the oven and bake for another 10 minutes, or until cheese is melted and bubbly.

Health Benefit: This pizza alternative provides a high protein content with the chicken crust and cheese, supporting muscle repair and growth.

36. Steak and Eggs

Prep Time: 5 minutes

Cook Time: 10 minutes

Ingredients:

- 1 8-oz sirloin steak

- 2 eggs

- Salt to taste

Preparation Instructions:

1. Season the steak with salt and cook to your preferred doneness in a skillet over medium-high heat, about 4-5 minutes per side for medium-rare.
2. In another pan, fry the eggs to your liking.
3. Serve the steak sliced with eggs on the side.

Health Benefit: Combines high-quality proteins and fats, essential for hormone balance and sustaining energy levels throughout the day.

37. Baked Whole Chicken

Prep Time: 10 minutes
Cook Time: 1 hour 30 minutes
Ingredients:

- 1 whole chicken (about 4 lbs)
- Salt to taste

Preparation Instructions:

1. Preheat your oven to 375°F (190°C).
2. Pat the chicken dry with paper towels and season inside and out with salt.
3. Place in a roasting pan and bake for about 1.5 hours, or until the internal temperature reaches 165°F (74°C).

Health Benefit: Provides a variety of proteins from different parts of the chicken, including collagen-rich parts like the skin, beneficial for joint and skin health.

38. Lamb Shank

Prep Time: 5 minutes
Cook Time: 2 hours

Ingredients:
  - 2 lamb shanks
  - Salt to taste

Preparation Instructions:
  1. Preheat your oven to 325°F (163°C).
  2. Season lamb shanks with salt.
  3. Roast in a covered dish for 2 hours, or until the meat is tender and falls off the bone.

Health Benefit:
Lamb is a good source of iron, zinc, and B vitamins, supporting immune function and energy levels.

39. Bacon Omelette

Prep Time: 5 minutes

Cook Time: 10 minutes

Ingredients:

- 3 eggs

- 4 slices of bacon, chopped

- Salt to taste

Preparation Instructions:

1. Cook bacon in a skillet until crispy. Remove and set aside.
2. Beat eggs with salt and pour into the skillet with bacon fat.
3. Add the crispy bacon pieces, cook until the omelette is set, fold, and serve.

Health Benefit: Offers a rich source of protein and fats from both eggs and bacon, supporting sustained energy and satiety.

40. Deviled Eggs

Prep Time: 15 minutes

Cook Time: 10 minutes

Ingredients:

- 6 eggs

- 1/4 cup mayonnaise

- Salt to taste

Preparation Instructions:

1. Hard boil the eggs, cool, peel, and halve them.

2. Scoop out the yolks and mix with mayonna ise and salt until smooth.

3. Pipe or spoon the yolk mixture back into the egg white halves.

Health Benefit: Eggs are a great source of choline, which is important for brain health and liver function.

41. Pork Loin Roast

Prep Time: 10 minutes

Cook Time: 1 hour

Ingredients:

- 2 lb pork loin roast
- Salt to taste

Preparation Instructions:

1. Preheat your oven to 375°F (190°C).

2. Season the pork loin all over with salt.

3. Roast in the oven for about 1 hour, or until the internal temperature reaches 145°F (63°C).

4. Let it rest for 10 minutes before slicing.

Health Benefit: Pork loin is a lean protein source, providing essential nutrients for muscle maintenance and overall health, without excessive fat.

42. Grilled Quail

Prep Time: 5 minutes
Cook Time: 15 minutes

Ingredients:
- 4 quails, cleaned and prepared
- Salt to taste

Preparation Instructions:
1. Preheat your grill to medium-high heat.
2. Season the quails inside and out with salt.
3. Grill for about 7-8 minutes per side, or until the meat is cooked through and the skin is crispy.

Health Benefit:
Quail provides a high-quality protein and is rich in vitamins and minerals like iron, supporting energy levels and healthy circulation.

43. Chicken Drumsticks

Prep Time: 5 minutes

Cook Time: 40 minutes

Ingredients:

- 6 chicken drumsticks
- Salt to taste

Preparation Instructions:

1. Preheat your oven to 400°F (200°C).
2. Season drumsticks with salt and place on a baking sheet.
3. Bake for 40 minutes, or until the skin is crispy and the meat is cooked through.

Health Benefit:

Chicken drumsticks are a good source of protein, niacin, and selenium, which are important for energy metabolism and antioxidant defense.

44. Egg Salad

Prep Time: 10 minutes

Cook Time: 10 minutes

Ingredients:

- 6 hard-boiled eggs, peeled and chopped

- 1/4 cup mayonnaise

- Salt to taste

Preparation Instructions:

1. Combine the chopped eggs with mayonnaise and salt in a bowl. Mix well.
2. Adjust seasoning to taste and serve chilled.

Health Benefit: Eggs are a complete protein source, providing all nine essential amino acids necessary for the human body, supporting tissue repair and muscle growth.

45. Pan-Seared Foie Gras

Prep Time: 5 minutes

Cook Time: 5 minutes

Ingredients:

- 4 slices of foie gras, about 1/2 inch thick

- Salt to taste

Preparation Instructions:

1. Season the foie gras slices with salt.
2. Heat a dry skillet over medium-high heat. Once hot, sear the foie gras for about 2 minutes per side.
3. Serve immediately.

Health Benefit: Foie gras is rich in vitamins A and B12, supporting vision health and energy metabolism.

46. Beef Short Ribs

Prep Time: 10 minutes

Cook Time: 3 hours

Ingredients:

- 4 beef short ribs
- Salt to taste

Preparation Instructions:

1. Preheat your oven to 300°F (150°C).
2. Season the short ribs with salt and place in a baking dish.
3. Cover with foil and bake for about 3 hours, or until the meat is tender and falls off the bone.

Health Benefit: Beef is a great source of high-quality protein, zinc, and iron, important for immune function and oxygen transport.

47. Butter-Basted Lobster Tails

Prep Time: 5 minutes

Cook Time: 10 minutes

Ingredients:

- 2 lobster tails

- 1/4 cup butter

- Salt to taste

Preparation Instructions:

1. Preheat your broiler.

2. Split the lobster tails down the middle, season with salt, and place a piece of butter on top of each.

3. Broil for about 10 minutes, or until the meat is opaque and cooked through.

Health Benefit:

Lobster is low in fat and high in protein and selenium, supporting thyroid function and cardiovascular health.

48. Carnivore Beef Stew

Prep Time: 10 minutes

Cook Time: 2 hours

Ingredients:

- 2 lbs beef chuck, cut into chunks

- 1/4 cup beef tallow

- Salt to taste

Preparation Instructions:

1. Heat the tallow in a large pot over medium-high heat.

2. Season the beef chunks with salt and brown in the tallow.

3. Add water just to cover the beef, bring to a simmer, then reduce heat and cover.

4. Cook for about 2 hours, or until the beef is tender.

Health Benefit:

This stew is rich in protein, fats, and collagen, which can help support joint health and skin elasticity.

49. Crispy Fried Fish

Prep Time: 5 minutes

Cook Time: 10 minutes

Ingredients:

- 4 fish fillets

- 1/4 cup lard or tallow for frying

- Salt to taste

Preparation Instructions:

1. Season the fish fillets with salt.
2. Heat the lard or tallow in a skillet over medium-high heat.
3. Fry the fish for about 5 minutes per side, or until golden and crispy.

Health Benefit:

Fish is an excellent source of omega-3 fatty acids and protein, promoting heart health and muscle maintenance.

50. Ground Lamb Skillet

Prep Time: 5 minutes

Cook Time: 10 minutes

Ingredients:

- 1 lb ground lamb
- Salt to taste

Preparation Instructions:

1. Heat a skillet over medium-high heat.
2. Add the ground lamb and season with salt. Cook, breaking apart with a spoon, until browned and cooked through.
3. Serve hot.

Health Benefit:

Lamb is a good source of omega-3 fatty acids, protein, and essential nutrients like zinc and vitamin B12, supporting brain health and immune function.

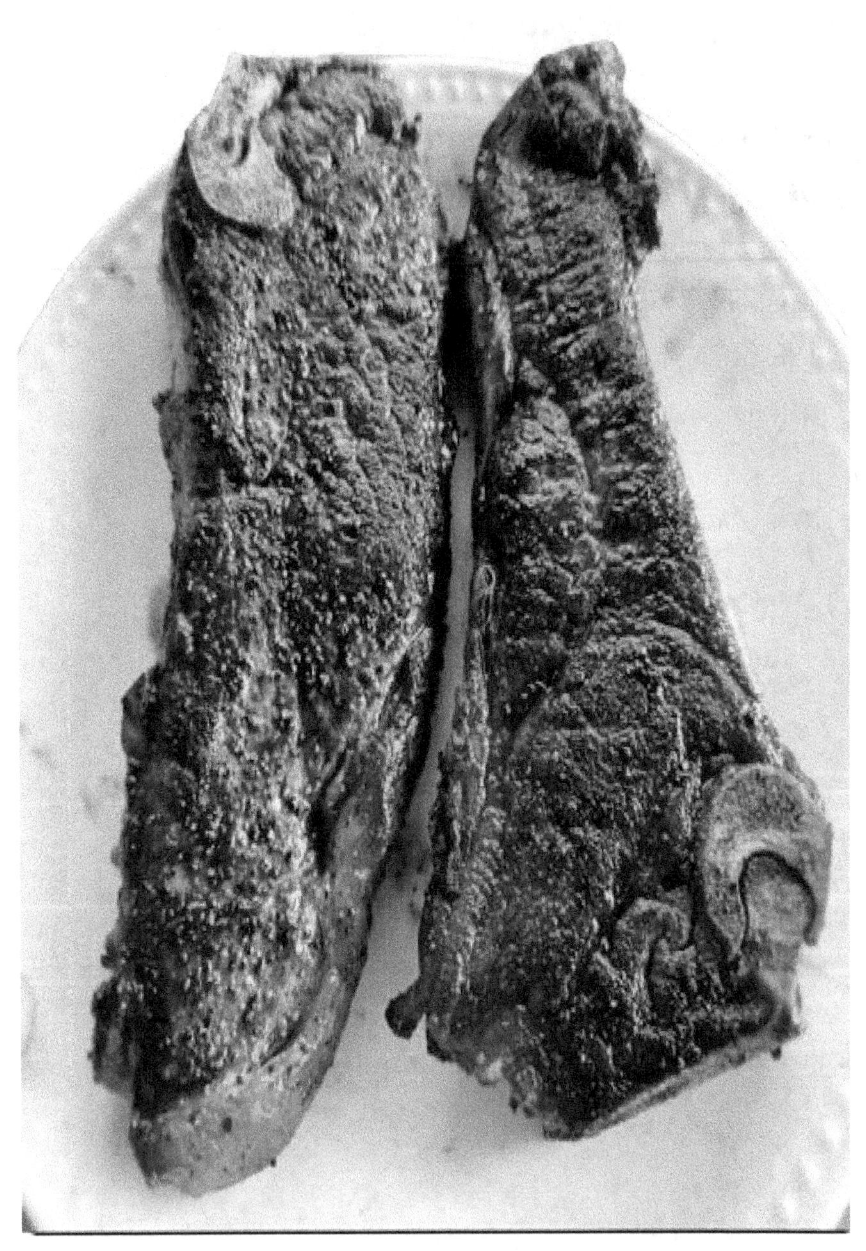

3. A FLEXIBLE 14-DAY CARNIVORE DIET MEAL PLAN FOR WOMEN

Day 1

- Breakfast: Bacon and Egg Frittata (8)

- Lunch: Classic Beef Steak (1)

- Dinner: Baked Pork Chops (3)

Day 2

- Breakfast: Scrambled Eggs with Cheese (14)

- Lunch: Grilled Ribeye Steak (9)

- Dinner: Roasted Turkey Legs (17)

Day 3

- Breakfast: Egg Muffins with Ham (28)

- Lunch: Seared Lamb Ribs (4)

- Dinner: Butter-Basted Chicken Breast (22)

Day 4

- Breakfast: Carnivore "Pizza" (35)

- Lunch: Bison Burger (31)

- Dinner: Pan-Fried Fish Fillets (19)

Day 5

- Breakfast: Bacon Omelette (39)

- Lunch: Chicken Drumsticks (43)

- Dinner: Slow-Cooked Beef Brisket (18)

Day 6

- Breakfast: Deviled Eggs (40)

- Lunch: Beef Short Ribs (46)

- Dinner: Grilled Sardines (26)

Day 7

- Breakfast: Pork Sausage Patties (29)

- Lunch: Venison Steaks (32)

- Dinner: Crispy Chicken Thighs (2)

Day 8

- Breakfast: Bacon and Egg Muffins (9, modified to use muffin tins)

- Lunch: Beef Bone Broth (11) with shredded Beef Steak (1)

- Dinner: Grilled Quail (42)

Day 9

- Breakfast: Carnivore Meatballs (21)

- Lunch: Smoked Trout (34)

- Dinner: Butter-Basted Lobster Tails (47)

Day 10

- Breakfast: Egg Salad (44)

- Lunch: Pork Loin Roast (41)

- Dinner: Bacon-Wrapped Shrimp (33)

Day 11

- Breakfast: Pork Rind Pancakes (35, modified with pork rinds)

- Lunch: Roasted Bone Marrow (27)

- Dinner: Baked Ham (23)

Day 12

- Breakfast: Carnivore Scotch Eggs (8, modified to use sausage meat)

- Lunch: Duck Breast (15)

- Dinner: Carnivore Beef Stew (48)

Day 13

- Breakfast: Steak and Eggs (36)

- Lunch: Crispy Fried Fish (49)

- Dinner: Baked Whole Chicken (37)

Day 14

- Breakfast: Ground Lamb Skillet (50)

- Lunch: Chicken Liver Pâté (7) on Crispy Chicken Skins (16)

- Dinner: Pan-Seared Foie Gras (45)

This meal plan is carefully crafted to offer a wide range of delicious animal-based foods that are packed with nutrients. It is specifically tailored to support the overall health of women following a carnivore diet. It is crucial to customize portion sizes and ingredients based on personal health requirements, preferences, and dietary objectives.

Also, seeking guidance from a healthcare provider or a nutritionist, particularly when adhering to a specialized diet, can help ensure that nutritional requirements are met in a safe and effective manner.

4. CONCLUSION

As we reach the end of the "Carnivore Diet Cookbook for Women," it becomes evident that this experience goes beyond just our meals. It's a joyful exploration of reclaiming our natural power, energy, and well-being through the nourishment that Mother Nature offers. This cookbook has been your trusted guide in discovering the ease and flavor of a carnivore diet, providing recipes that not only please your taste buds but also provide the essential nutrients your body needs, tailored specifically for women.

Adopting a carnivore lifestyle is a personal decision that many women find empowering. It's all about tuning in to your body, comprehending its requirements, and providing it with nourishment that empowers you. The recipes in this book, from the invigorating breakfasts to the fulfilling dinners, have been carefully crafted to assist you on your journey, supplying the necessary nutrients for hormonal balance, bone density, mental clarity, and much more.

As you progress on your journey, keep in mind that the essence of this diet is about quality, simplicity, and paying attention to your body's cues. Many women have discovered the transformative power of the carnivore diet, which goes beyond being a temporary regimen and becomes a sustainable and enriching way of life. It's all about getting back to the fundamentals, embracing the nourishment that nature offers, and celebrating the multitude of health benefits that come with it.

We trust that this cookbook has sparked your creativity, introduced exciting tastes to your meals, and supported your path to better health and overall wellness. May these recipes serve as a tribute to the incredible women who nourish their bodies and minds with strength and resilience. Cheers to your well-being, energy, and the happiness that comes from adopting a lifestyle that is both nourishing and satisfying. Keep discovering, savoring, and flourishing on your carnivore diet journey.

HAPPY

COOKING!

www.ingramcontent.com/pod-product-compliance
Lightning Source LLC
Chambersburg PA
CBHW070813250726
48662CB00004B/2037